✓ S0-BYF-599

unique
A W F #L G5 ✓

A BEGINNER'S GUIDE TO

Shiatsu

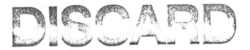

USING JAPANESE FINGER PRESSURE FOR THE RELIEF OF HEADACHES, BACK PAIN, AND HYPERTENSION

DISCARD

Patrick McCarty

g 106877

Avery Publishing Group

Garden City Park, New York

SHELBYVILLE-SHELBY COUNTY
PUBLIC LIBRARY

The medical and health procedures in this book are based on training, personal experiences, and research of the author. Because each person and situation is unique, the editor and the publisher urge the reader to check with a qualified health professional before using any procedure where there is any question as to its appropriateness.

The publisher does not advocate the use of any particular diet or exercise program but believes the information presented in this book should be available to the public.

Because there is always some risk involved, the author and publisher are not responsible for any adverse effects or consequences resulting from the use of any of the suggestions, preparations, or procedures in this book. Please do not use the book if you are unwilling to assume the risk. Feel free to consult a physician or other qualified health professional. It is a sign of wisdom, not cowardice, to seek a second or third opinion.

Cover Design: William Gonzalez
Cover Photograph: Tony Stone Images
Interior Illustrations: Susan Reid
Printer: Paragon Press, Honesdale, PA

Cataloging-in-Publication Data

McCarty, Patrick, 1947-
    Beginners guide to shiatsu : relieving headaches, back pain, and hypertension with japanese finger pressure / by Patrick McCarty.
    p.cm.
    Includes index.
    Originally published: Eureka, CA: Turning Point, 1986.
    ISBN 0-89529-659-4

    1. Acupressure I. Title
    RM723.A27M33 1995   615.8'22
                                         QB195-220

Copyright © 1995 by Patrick McCarty.

All rights reserved. No part of this publication may be reproduced, stored in retrieval system, or transmitted, in any form or by any means, electronic mechanical, photocopying, recording or otherwise, without the prior written consent of the copyright owner.

Printed in the United States of America

10 9 8 7 6 5 4 3 2 1

Contents

To Meredith

for the love and nourishment she gives.

Introduction

Over the last several years I have had the good fortune to meet and work with many interesting people here in the U.S., Japan, China, Latin America and Europe. In these places, I have either taught shiatsu classes or given treatments in this unique massage form. From this exchange between friends I have learned much more than I have taught. But isn't that the purpose of teaching? Not only have I learned about the techniques of shiatsu and its effectiveness. I have learned about life. Massage has a way of bringing you into contact with others. It also is an effective way to know yourself.

My studies and collaboration with Shizuko Yamamoto, one of the world's foremost natural health consultants and originator of "Barefoot Shiatsu", has set my direction in therapy to follow the Way of Nature. Together with my study of traditional Chinese medicine in the People's Republic of China and work with Ms. Yamamoto, my interest has been guided to emphasize preventive healing practices. Practices that place the individual as an integral part of nature. Without this fundamental understanding true healing will escape us.

The purpose of this manual is to serve as a basic guide to Barefoot Shiatsu. For those who have taken a shiatsu course it will act as a reminder of both the spirit and technique of shiatsu. For the many who have not yet participated in classes this book can serve as a step-by-step guide, and hopefully stimulate your interest so that sometime you will want to continue your studies in this unique art form.

Without nature we could not exist. It is the simple things in nature that bring the greatest joy. Shiatsu follows the way of nature. Practiced with the right spirit, shiatsu can bring us all health and happiness. It is my hope that this will happen for you.

Theory of Shiatsu and Preventive Health Care

When someone is hurting either physically or emotionally our human instinct is to reach out and comfort that person. We automatically want to touch. This intuitive response is the foundation of massage. We aren't trying to medically treat the person we are just trying to comfort them; and ease the pain. It is important to remember when practicing shiatsu that our instincts come first and our techniques follow. Given the proper attitude of caring, the technique will always naturally develop. With the trial and error of thousands of years of experience, it is easy to see how a systematic approach to touch has evolved. This system is shiatsu.

In Japanese the word "shi" means finger and "atsu" means pressure. Shiatsu, also called Acupressure, is an Oriental healing method in which specific points on the body surface are pressed with the fingers. An outgrowth of the ancient traditional medicine practiced in China, shiatsu was brought to Japan in the sixth century. Presently it is recognized in Japan as a valuable medical aid.

Chinese medicine views a healthy body as one in which life energy is balanced and flowing freely through fourteen invisible channels called meridians. Twelve channels are directly connected with the body's internal organs, while two channels deal with important circulatory functions. When vital energy becomes imbalanced (too weak or too strong) or stagnated in the channels, the body develops troubles; vitality drops and discomfort and sickness may occur.

Energy tends to stagnate in specific points along the channels called acupoints. There are hundreds of acupoints in the

2

human body. When energy is blocked in an acupoint, it becomes sensitive to pressure. In shiatsu the acupoints are pressed to stimulate the movement of stagnated energy as well as to diagnose the presence of disease.

The presence of illness serves as a warning from nature that tells us of our error. In some way nature is being violated. The symptoms of illness are protective mechanisms. If we listen and heed the warning then further development is avoided. In other words if we pay attention to natural signals many illnesses will be prevented.

Shiatsu never cures the patient. It is the patient who heals himself. The practitioner is the stimulus to aid the patient in assuming a proper direction. The practitioner serves as a mirror for the patient, allowing the patient the opportunity to self-reflect on the true cause of his or her condition. Our approach is educational.

Shiatsu creates a deep feeling of well-being, vitality and relaxation, and is an effective tool in preventing disease. It can eliminate muscular stiffness, reduce tensions, relieve fatigue, and strengthen the internal organs. Shiatsu can be a pleasurable experience. It encourages communication between family members, couples and friends. It requires no special equipment, oil or the removal of clothes. It can be done anywhere, at anytime.

Understanding Illness

From observing nature the theory of traditional natural healing has developed. The ancient Chinese teachers and physicians set up a medical system which patterned itself on nature's ways. It was discovered that everything is constantly changing. The changes were predictable and from this came the laws of Yin and Yang, the governing forces within the universe. The ancients saw that energy circulated in a distinct pattern from organ to organ within the body, the way a river flows within

3

it's banks on its voyage from the mountain to the sea. This vital energy moved from organ to organ animating each one, giving it the fuel to function.

Any obstruction of this flow in vital energy created problems. In order to cure the problem, balance had to be re-established.

1. LUNG

Channel-Yin   Organ-Yang
Energy Flow-Body to Hand   Active 3-5 am.

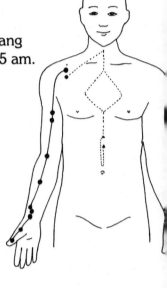

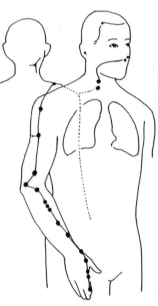

2. LARGE INTESTINE

Channel -Yang   Organ-Yin
Energy Flow-Hand   Active 5-7 am.
to Head

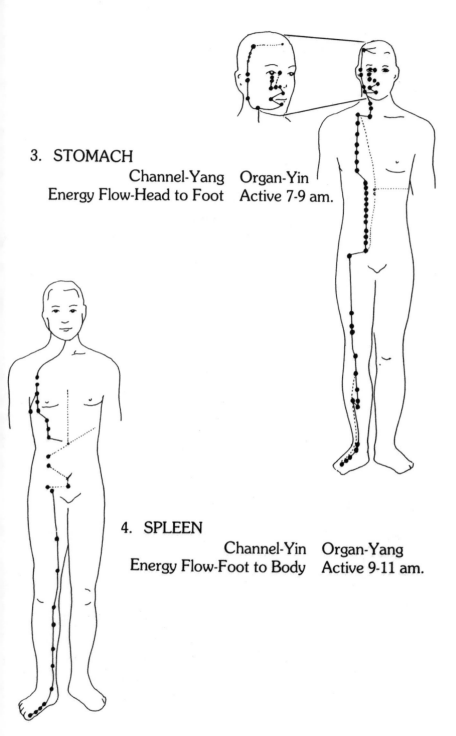

3. STOMACH

Channel-Yang   Organ-Yin
Energy Flow-Head to Foot   Active 7-9 am.

4. SPLEEN

Channel-Yin   Organ-Yang
Energy Flow-Foot to Body   Active 9-11 am.

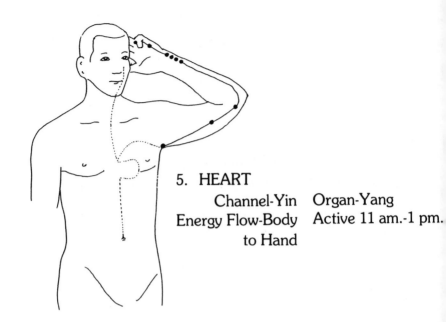

5. HEART

      Channel-Yin   Organ-Yang
Energy Flow-Body   Active 11 am.-1 pm.
        to Hand

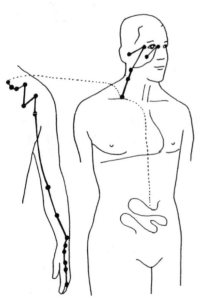

6. SMALL INTESTINE

Channel-Yang   Organ-Yin
  Energy Flow-   Active 1-3 pm.
Hand to Head

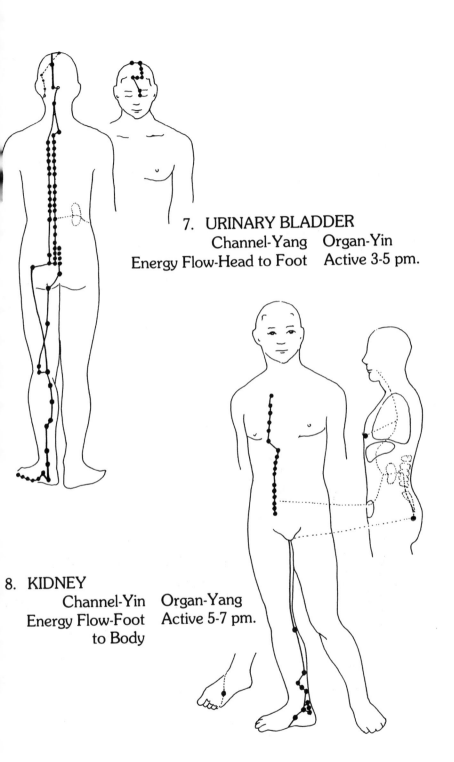

7. URINARY BLADDER
Channel-Yang   Organ-Yin
Energy Flow-Head to Foot   Active 3-5 pm.

8. KIDNEY
Channel-Yin   Organ-Yang
Energy Flow-Foot   Active 5-7 pm.
to Body

7

9. HEART GOVERNOR
Channel- Yin
Energy Flow-Body   Active 7-9 pm.
to Hand

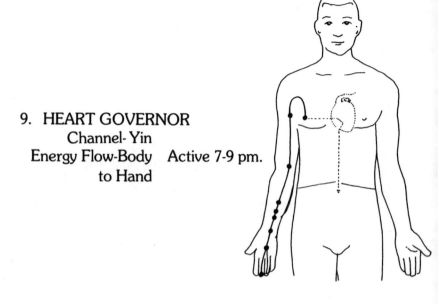

10. TRIPLE HEATER
Channel Yang
Energy Flow-   Active 9-11 pm.
Hand to Body

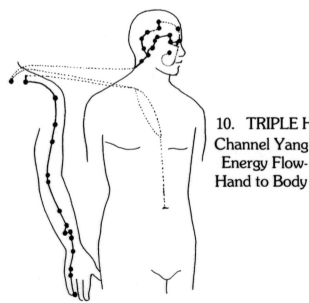

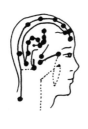

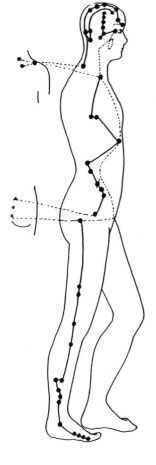

11. GALL BLADDER
Channel- Yang   Organ-Yin
Energy Flow-Head   Active 11 pm.-1 am.
to Foot

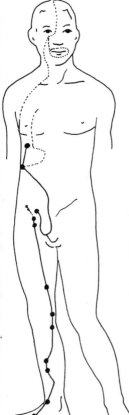

12. LIVER
Channel-Yin   Organ-Yang
Energy Flow-Foot to Body   Active 1-3 am.

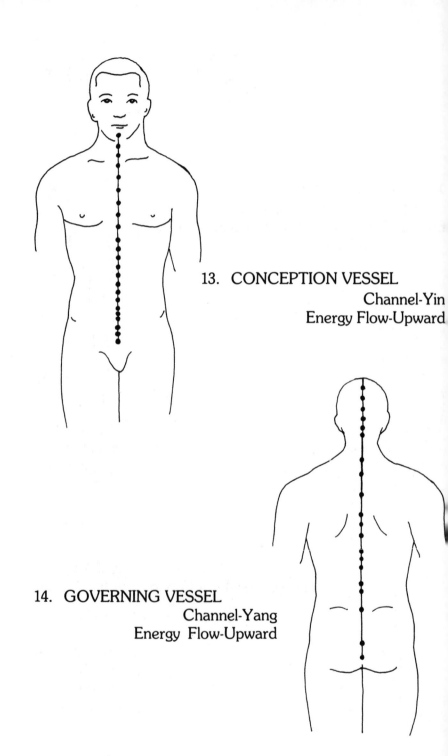

13. CONCEPTION VESSEL
Channel-Yin
Energy Flow-Upward

14. GOVERNING VESSEL
Channel-Yang
Energy Flow-Upward

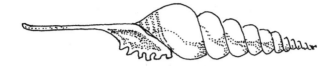

Yin and Yang

The universal symbol of yin and yang is the spiral. As everything in life is constantly changing, the direction of that change is either one way or another, moving inward or moving outward. Basic to the understanding of this principle is the assumption that the elements of nature are temporary and changing. These two forces are always opposite and antagonistic, and yet at the same time they are complementary, for they are always combining and cooperating.

All energy and influence that comes from outside the earth, that is from the sun, stars, constellations, infinite space, or what we think of as heaven's force, is called YANG. This yang force comes frc.n heaven toward the earth. Its movement is centripetal, that is from the periphery toward the center. Objects influenced by yang force are being contracted. They become smaller, harder and produce heat.

An opposite force comes from the earth. The earth's rotation produces a force that we call YIN. Its movement is centrifugal, that is from the center toward the periphery. This force causes objects to expand and become larger. They also become softer, less dense and produce coolness.

In traditional Chinese medicine the cause of illness is considered to be an imbalance between Yin and Yang. There are several important factors that create this imbalance. It is either one or a combination of the following which creates illness: external evil, internal evil or food.

External Evils

Cold - yin;   most appear in winter, damages the yang eg. fever.

Wind - yang;   always found with other symptoms - movable.

Damp - yin;   sluggish, blocks energy flow.

Heat - yang;   over perspiration, dehydration, short breath, cough, wheeze.

Dryness - yang in fall;   cracked lips, dry nose, sore throat.

Internal Evils

Joy (Excitability)	Heart	energy goes slow
Anger	Liver	energy goes up
Worry (thinking)	Spleen	blocks energy
Sadness	Lung	diminishes energy
Fear - Fright	Kidney	(fear-energy goes down)
		(fright-goes out of order)

Food

overeating

bad food - eg. oil and sugar cause damp which spoils the spleen

Foundation of Health

Our day-to-day activities are the foundation of our health. Within this realm is found the cause of our illness and strength. Looking into life's common activities will give us great insight into the fundamentals of health.

Movement

In the past everyone was much more physically active. Our present sedentary life with less and less movement allows problems to arise. Obesity, joint and muscle pain and weakness can be avoided with regular exercise.

Try to exercise 2-3 times per week, especially enough so that you work up a sweat. Fifteen to thirty minutes at a time is enough. In addition to being beneficial to the heart and vessel system, it helps to regulate the appetite.

Breathing

Never forget about your breathing while giving a shiatsu treatment. It is the breath that unifies the body and the mind. Breathing should come from the lower abdomen not from the chest. You will maintain stamina and have a more powerful treatment when your breathing is slow and deep. If you want to relax the receiver, have them exhale. When you want force and power, use the inhalation. Through proper use of the breath you can lead the receiver to a peaceful state of relaxation.

Diet

At every moment, a great many activities are taking place in all the millions of cells of the body. For these activities to go on there must be a regular supply of nutrients. When these nutrients are not provided in the proper balance by food, the body does not function at its best. The food that we eat exerts a major influence on how well our bodies function as well as health in general.

Our diet, like other aspects of life must conform to the principles of nature. If we eat the way people did thousands of years ago there will be no problem. However we have gotten away from our traditional eating patterns and are now faced with the fact that sixty percent of all illnesses are diet-related.

A diet rich in whole natural foods satisfies our biological needs. Within a diet high in whole cereal grains, beans, vegetables, seaweed, nuts, seeds and fruit, with occasional fish, can be found all the vitamins, minerals, carbohydrates, fats and protein as well as yet undiscovered necessities for well-being. The key to dietary health is to remember "whole and in-season". This will eliminate all unnecessary items such as sugar, beef, dairy products, refined and junk foods and chemicals used as additives.

Sex

The act of making love is necessary for life to continue. A healthy and satisfying sex life lays an important cornerstone in a marriage. Many problems find their basis in sex. Both excessive and non-existant sexual desire are symptoms that an imbalance exists in this aspect of life.

Sleep

No one has ever been reported to have died from either too much or not enough sleep. But how do you feel when you don't get enough sleep? Besides irritability, it has been found that work performance decreases. When you sleep too much it is easy to be depressed. Most people sleep between 6-8 hours.

Five Transformations

The inter-relatedness of all creation is represented in the Five Transformations. The natural elements of fire, earth, metal, water and wood are used to show the various stages that energy goes through endlessly. Within each stage there are distinct qualities. The following chart will familiarize you with these qualities. Fire is the creator or mother of earth. Earth is the son of Fire. The mother nourishes the son. If the son is in difficulty, talking with the mother can help the son. Stimulating the mother (fire) will help the son (earth). In turn each element is both at one time a child and then a parent. This phase of the transformation is called inter-promoting (parent-child).

When one element is too active it can have negative effects. For example if Water is hyperactive it will negatively affect Fire. Water (Kidney/Bladder) will put out the Fire (Heart/Small Intestine). This phase of energy transformation is called counter-acting.

The Five Transformations are a helpful tool which can unify and clarify formerly unknown relationships within the body. For example in the case of skin problems, we know that the skin is governed by the Lung. The season when the Lung receives a greater amount of universal energy is autumn. During autumn the lung and subsequently the skin has the greatest chance to be strengthened. The pungent flavor as found in horseradish or mustard, particularly effects the lung. The grain, vegetable and fruit which benefit this organ are brown rice, onion and peach.

Organ	Element	Season	Flavor	Grain	Veget
LU/LI	Metal	Fall	Pungent	Brown Rice	Onion
SP/ST	Earth	Late Summer	Sweet	Millet	Squash
HT/SI	Fire	Summer	Bitter	Corn	Scallio
KD/UB	Water	Winter	Salty	Aduki	Greens
LV/GB	Wood	Spring	Sour	Wheat	Leeks

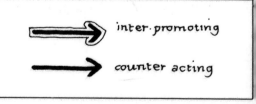

inter·promoting

counter acting

it	Governs	Humor	Motion	Emotion	Anatomy
ch	Skin and Body Hair	Runny eyes & nose	Cough	Melancholy	Nose
e	Flesh	Drooling	Hiccough, stutter	Anxiety, worry	Mouth
cot	Blood Vessels	Sweating	Excessive laughing & talking	Excitability	Tongue
stnut	Head Hair and Bones	Watery eyes	Clenched fists	Fear	Ear
n	Ligaments, saliva and muscles	Saliva	Trembling	Anger	Eyes

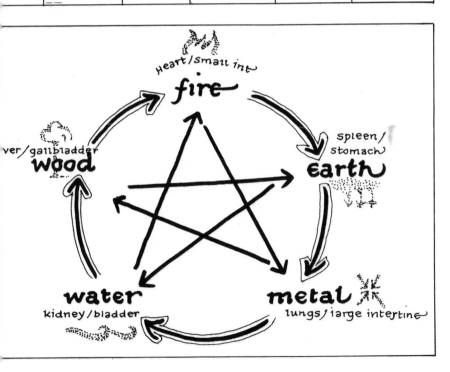

Understanding the Energy Channels

All channels either begin or end in the hands or feet. With manipulation we can bring about a change in the functioning of each channel system.

A continuous flow of energy passes from one channel system to the next. Beginning with the lung channel, energy passes to the large intestine channel. From there it continues on to the stomach channel. Eventually, it will pass through each part of the body and then begin to flow again within the lung channel.

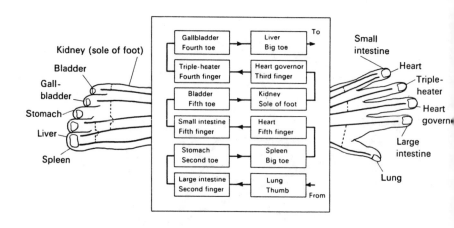

Complete Body Shiatsu

The most effective method to balance an individual's physical and mental energy is to give a complete shiatsu session. Shiatsu can be used as a "tune up" and as a preventive measure against illness. It is useful when you are feeling half-healthy. That is when you are tired and listless but no medical symptoms are present. You are not really sick but you're not well either. Shiatsu can also be used when specific illness is present such as hypertension, constipation, diabetes as well as the common cold, stiff neck and shoulders.

When you give a treatment here are some things to think about which will enhance the treatments effectiveness.

1. Use your breathing. Learn how to control it and use it in harmony with the receiver. When you want the receiver to relax emphasize the exhalation.

2. Find your balance. Find your balancing point and keep that center while you are giving the treatment.

3. Eat well. Keep yourself in good condition. The person receiving the session will be able to feel this.

4. Trust in nature. Give the best treatment that you can and let nature take care of the healing.

BACK SIDE

Seated-on the floor or in a chair.

1. Active hand is on the spine near the neck. Other hand is on the shoulder. Let the active hand run down the spine feeling the condition of the spine and back muscles. Mentally note idiosyncracies.

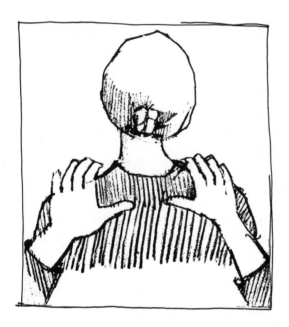

2. Loosen up the shoulders by randomly kneading and squeezing the shoulder muscles. The forefingers are over the shoulders with the thumbs on the back. Press with the thumbs, beginning near the spine working outward to the shoulder tips.

3. Do one shoulder blade at a time. One hand supports the opposite shoulder while the thumb presses around the contour made by the scapula on the back. While pressing with the thumbs the other fingers should still make contact with the shoulder.

4. With opposite hand do other contour of other shoulder blade.

5. Pound across the shoulders with fists or the side of the hand.

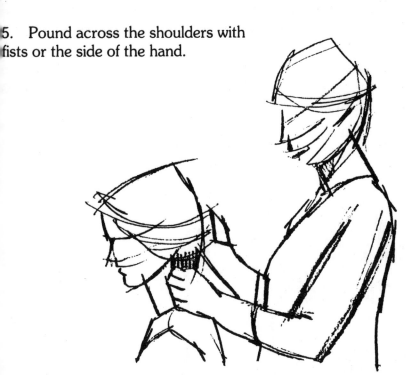

6. Go to the side. One hand supports the forehead. The other hand is placed on the back of the neck. One knee is placed in the middle of the back for support. (If the right hand is on the neck then it is the right knee that is used for support.) Squeeze and knead the neck with the fingers and thumb.

7. With the thumb press the muscles of the side of the neck. Press from under the ear to the shoulder.

8. Change to the receiver's other side. Support the forehead, neck and back then press the side of the neck with the other hand.

9. Find the indentation in the middle of the back of the neck. Place your thumb there. Have the receiver breath in and on an exhalation gently rock the head back onto the thumb and hold for three seconds. Repeat three times. Use your body weight.

10. Stand in back of the receiver and press across the top of the shoulders with your thumbs. Begin in the center and press outward. Repeat several times.

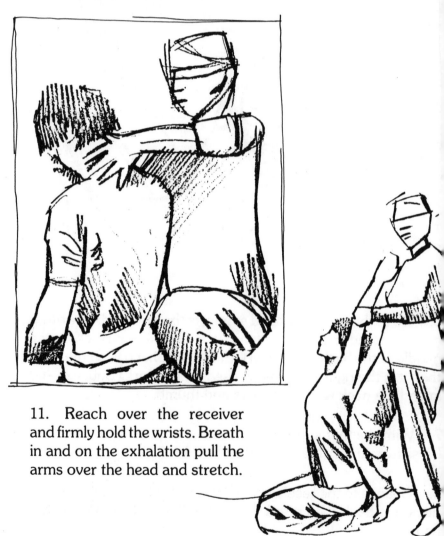

11. Reach over the receiver and firmly hold the wrists. Breath in and on the exhalation pull the arms over the head and stretch.

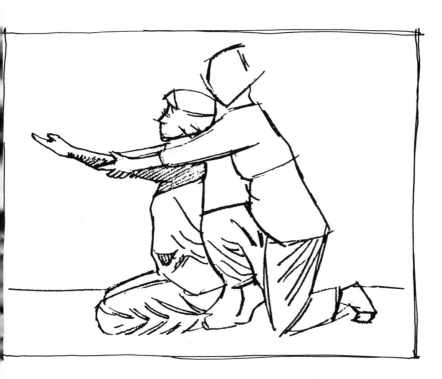

12. Hold the arms at the elbows, on an exhalation have the receiver bring the head back while you pull the elbow back, stretching between the shoulder blades.

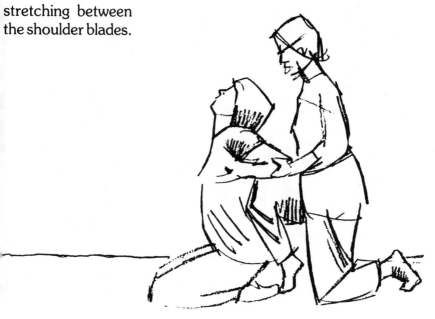

23

LYING FACE DOWN

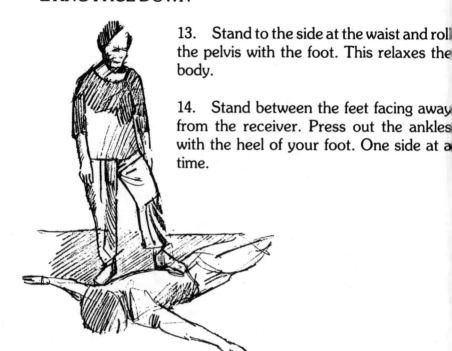

13.   Stand to the side at the waist and roll the pelvis with the foot. This relaxes the body.

14.   Stand between the feet facing away from the receiver. Press out the ankles with the heel of your foot. One side at a time.

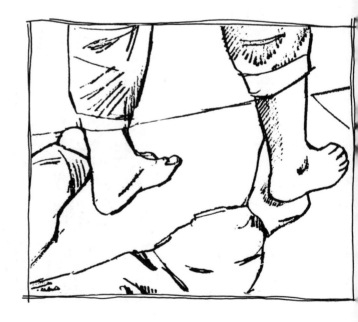

24

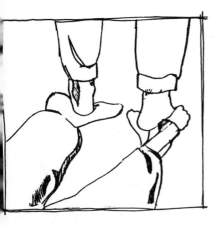

15. Walk down the feet. Your toes on the floor support your weight while the heels press the bottom of the receiver's feet.

16. Stand to the right side. With the foot closest to the receiver's foot, adjust the achilles tendon.

17. With the ball or heel of your foot gently press from the ankle up to just below the knee. Repeat this several times. Never step on the knee.

18. Switch feet and press the buttock and the upper right thigh coming down to just above the knee. Repeat several times.

19. Go to other side and stand at knee. Repeat #16, 17, and 18.

20. Stand between the receiver's legs facing the head, stimulate with your foot the buttock region and the coccyx bone. Press along the inside of the thigh. Stimulation of the tail bone relaxes the autonomic nervous system.

SHELBYVILLE-SHELBY COUNTY
PUBLIC LIBRARY

21. Bend receiver's knees so feet are perpendicular to the floor. Wrap your fingers around the toes. Breath in, on an exhalation press the legs toward the buttocks.

22. Same position breath in and, on exhalation, cross legs and press down toward the buttocks.

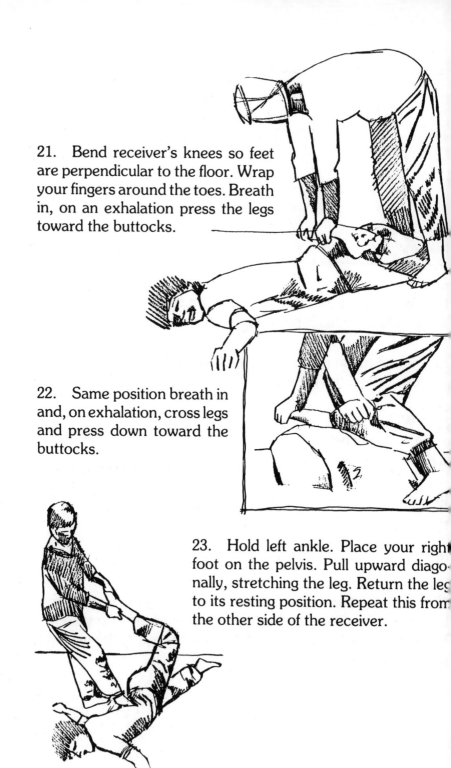

23. Hold left ankle. Place your right foot on the pelvis. Pull upward diagonally, stretching the leg. Return the leg to its resting position. Repeat this from the other side of the receiver.

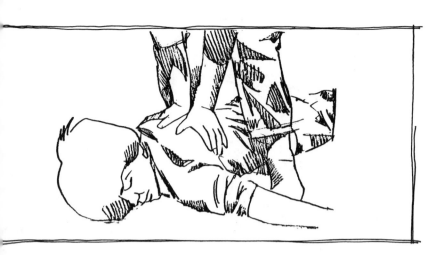

BACK SHIATSU

24. Stand astride the receiver. Place the wrist of your hands together and press directly on top of the spine between the shoulder blades. Your fingers should be pointing out toward the arms. Have the receiver breath in and on exhalation press straight down. Continue down to the waist.

25. If you have confidence then you can try this technique. If you use your common sense and are careful you will not have any problems. Use a chair for balance. Step up on the buttocks near the waist with most of your weight. With one foot near the waist bone use the other foot to press gently and loosen the back. Press the spine from the neck down to the waist. Remember that most of your weight remains on the hip and the chair.

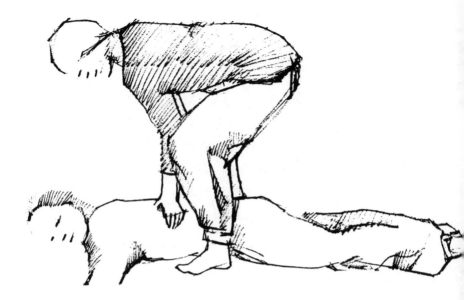

26. Stand with feet astride the receiver and knead th shoulders.

27. Place the thumbs close to the spine at the shoulder leve Co-ordinate your breathing with the receiver - that is breath i and out together. On an exhalation press the back leaning you body weight into it. Go slow and deep with a quick release at th end. Your back should be straight with your arms brace against your legs. Hold each point for 3-5 seconds. Move dow one vertebrae at a time until you reach the sacrum. Re- peat this line.

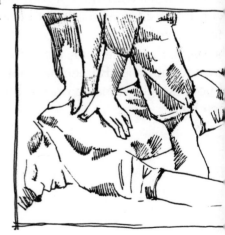

28. Same position and same technique but out three inches from the spine. Lean your body weight into each point. Start near the shoulders and continue until the sacrum, with coordinated breath.

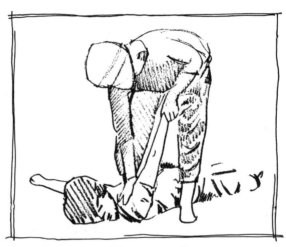

29. Place your right hand at the receiver's left shoulder. With the left hand take the receiver's left wrist and lift it, stretching the arm. Rotate it several times in both directions.

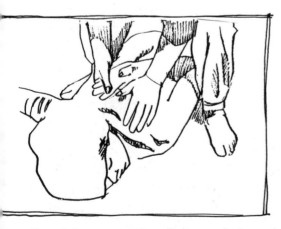

30. Bend the arm at the elbow and place the receiver's hand as far up on the back as is comfortable. Change hands. Hold the receiver's left hand with your right hand. With the left hand on the shoulder blade, lean your body weight on this blade.

31.   Press the contour of the shoulder blade with your thumb.

32.   Make an adjustment by pushing the arm upward toward the back of the neck.

33.   Change sides and stimulate the right arm by repeating #29, 30, 31, and 32.

34.   Kneel at the side. With loose fists, pound the back. You can also pound by holding your hands palm to palm and lightly striking with the back side of your hand.

FRONT SIDE

35.   Have receiver turn over onto the back. Stand at feet. Have the receiver bend knees up. Keeping knees together press down toward the abdomen. Rotate in one direction and then the other.

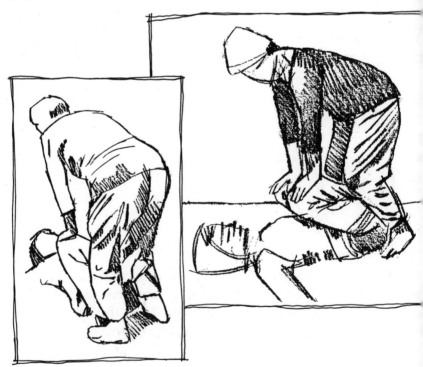

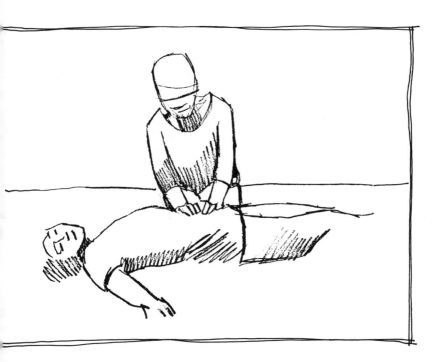

Abdomen

36.   Kneel on receiver's right side. With the hand, lightly probe the entire abdominal area, exploring each internal organ.

37.   With the heel of the hand rub in a clockwise direction.

38.   Knead the abdomen by pushing with the palm and pulling with the finger-tips. Somewhat like kneading bread. Do this for ten to fifteen cycles.

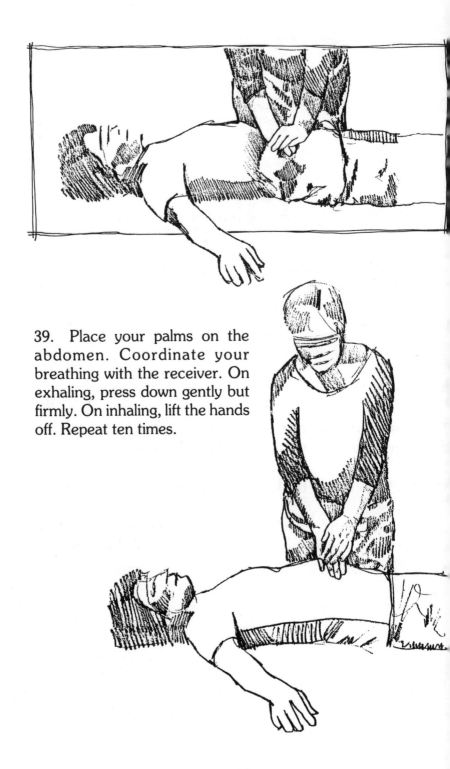

39. Place your palms on the abdomen. Coordinate your breathing with the receiver. On exhaling, press down gently but firmly. On inhaling, lift the hands off. Repeat ten times.

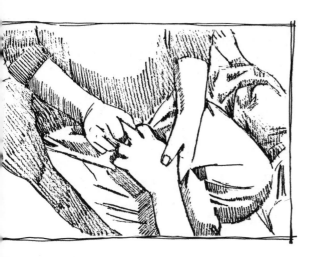

HANDS AND ARMS

0.   Still kneeling, pick up the receiver's right hand. Pull and stretch the arm toward yourself to loosen it. Hold the wrist with your inside hand (right) and with your outside hand (left) manipulate each finger beginning with the little one. Press both top and bottom and side to side. Press from where the wrist bends to each finger tip.

1.   Inside hand holds the wrist while the outside hand's fingers interlock with the receiver's. Bend the wrist back toward the body, stretching the fingers.

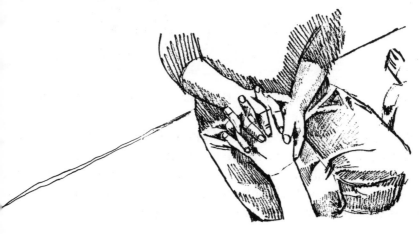

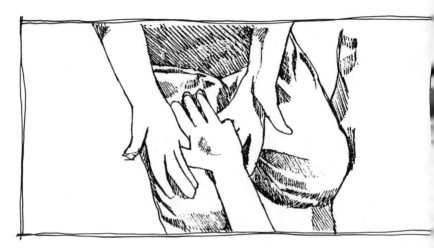

42.   Turn the palm up. Place the little finger of your right hand
between the receiver's little finger and ring finger. Place the little
finger of your left hand between your friend's index finger and
thumb. Spread and stretch the palm open.

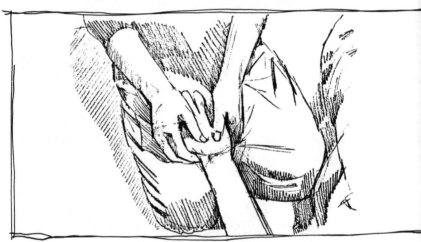

43.   In this position, press the palm area with your thumbs.

44.   Inside hand holds wrist. With your left hand, beginning at
the wrist, press upward directly above the index finger on the
bone to the elbow. Simultaneously on the bottom side of the
same arm press the index finger against that part of the arm. In
this way you are pressing two channels at once.

45. For the second line of the arm the hand positions are the same. Beginning at the same place near the wrist press up on a diagonal up to the elbow. As before the index finger is pressing from the underside, thus stimulating two channels.

46. Change hands. Left hand holds wrist. Right thumb presses directly up the center of the forearm. At the same time the index finger is pressing the center of the backside of the arm.

47. Change hands. Inside hand holds either hand or elbow. Outside hand presses from center of shoulder bone down to elbow.

48. Same hand press center of arm pit along inside of arm to elbow.

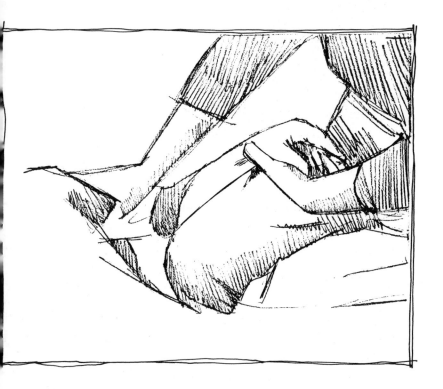

35

SHELBYVILLE-SHELBY COUNTY
PUBLIC LIBRARY

49.   Third line pressed is midway between first two. Each line is pressed several times.

50.   Grasp both hands around arm at bicep and squeeze, moving down to elbow and wrist.

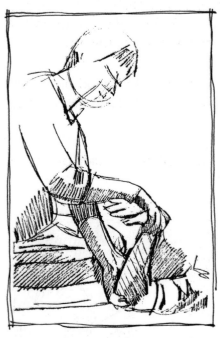

51.   Adjust arm by bending it and pulling it outward.

FEET AND LEGS

52.   Kneel at feet. Pick up both feet and sway back and forth to relax.

53.   Hold right foot with inside hand (right) and brush the toes with the outside hand (left).

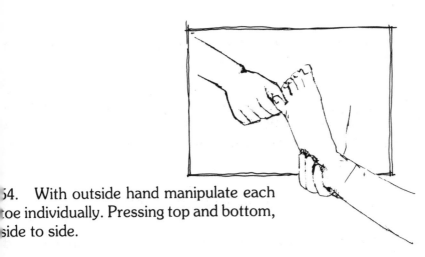

54.   With outside hand manipulate each
toe individually. Pressing top and bottom,
side to side.

55.   With the thumb press the bottom of the foot thoroughly.

56.   With outside hand press up shin bone from ankle to just
below the knee. Repeat several times.

57.   Same hand press up the inside of the leg from ankle to just
below the knee. Repeat several times.

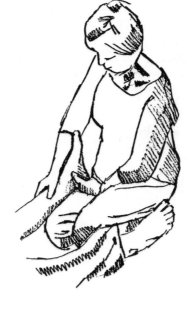

58.   Same hand. Outside fingers press around the bone on the outside of the leg. Repeat several times.

59.   Change hands. Inside hand holds foot. Outside hand (left) thumb presses near the bone on the muscle on the outside of the leg. Press from the ankle up to just below the knee. Repeat several times.

60.   Squeeze the calf muscle with the hand.

61.   Slightly bend the knee and pull the leg toward yourself and place on floor.

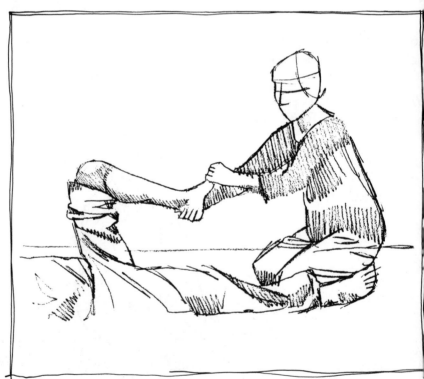

52. Pick up left leg with inside hand. Brush toes. Manipulate each toe. Press bottom of foot. Press shin bone, inside leg and outside leg. Change hands. Press outside leg. Squeeze calf muscle. (See #53-61) Bend knee and pull out leg stretch.

53. Go to left hand and arm. Repeat hand and arm treatment. Shake arm. Manipulate each finger. Interlock fingers and stretch. Press palm with thumbs. Press channels on top of arm. Second line on diagonal. Change hands. Press up center of forearm. Press upper arm on outside, arm pit and midway. Repeat each channel several times. Squeeze whole arm with hands. Adjust arm. (See #40-51)

HEAD AND FACE

54. Move to behind receiver's head. Lift the head and place chin on chest, stretching neck.

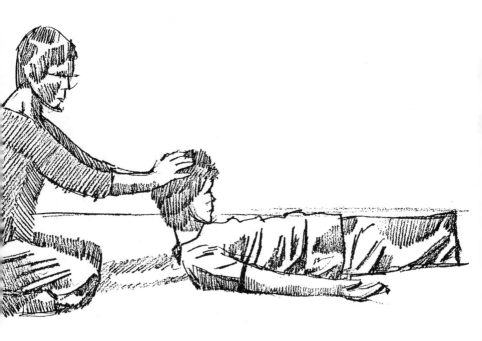

65.   Turn head to right side holding with right hand. Thumb presses the neck muscles from below ear to shoulder. Repeat several times.

66.   Turn head and press neck on other side.

67.   Index fingers press inside corners of the eyes.

68.   Press around eyes on rims both upper and lower. Beginning on inside working outward.

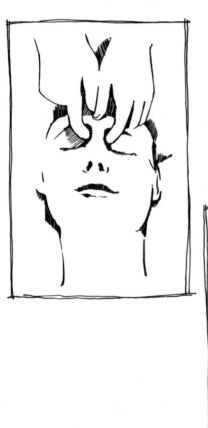

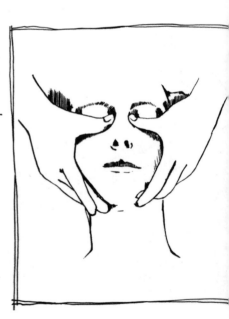

69.   Thumbs press temples. Hold for 2-5 seconds.

70.   Press down sides of nose and points at base of nose.

71.   Press above upper lip and around mouth.

72.   Thumbs on face and fingers under jaw press from the center back to the ear following jaw bone.

73.   Massage whole face with thumbs, increasing circulation.

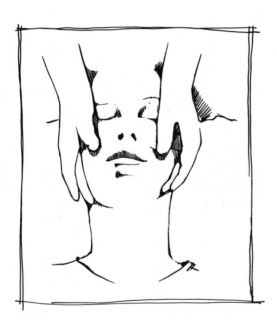

74.   With thumbs press a line from inside corners of eye brow over the forehead back into the hair.

75.   Place thumbs one on the other and press directly on the midline of the head from the center of the head to the point between the eyes. Repeat #74 and 75.

76.   Gently pull hair.

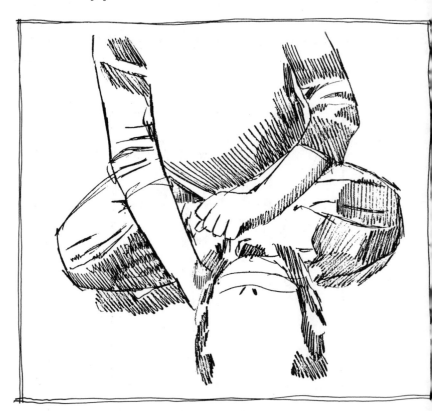

77.   Lightly pound the top and side of the head with the side of your hand or with a fist.

78.   Place the left hand on the forehead and the right hand on the neck and hold for fifteen seconds to one minute. Breathing with the receiver.

Acupoints Regulating Internal Functions

The Back-Shu acupoints relate to yang and can be used to treat internal diseases as well as diseases of the sense organs which are related to their respective corresponding internal organ. For example, UB 18 (T9), Liver, may be chosen to treat eye disorders, as the eye is the window of the liver. UB 13 - Lung, can be used to treat disorders of the nose. UB 15 - Heart, can be used to treat disorders of the tongue. UB 20 - Spleen, can be used to treat disorders of the mouth. UB 23 - Kidney, can be used to treat disorders of the ears and hearing.

Internal Organ	Acupoint	Location
Lung	UB 13	T3
Heart Governor	UB 14	T4
Heart	UB 15	T5
Liver	UB 18	T9
Gall Bladder	UB 19	T10
Spleen	UB 20	T11
Stomach	UB 21	T12
Three Heater	UB 22	L1
Kidney	UB 23	L2
Large Intestine	UB 25	L4
Small Intestine	UB 27	S1
Bladder	UB 28	S2

DIGESTIVE ORGANS

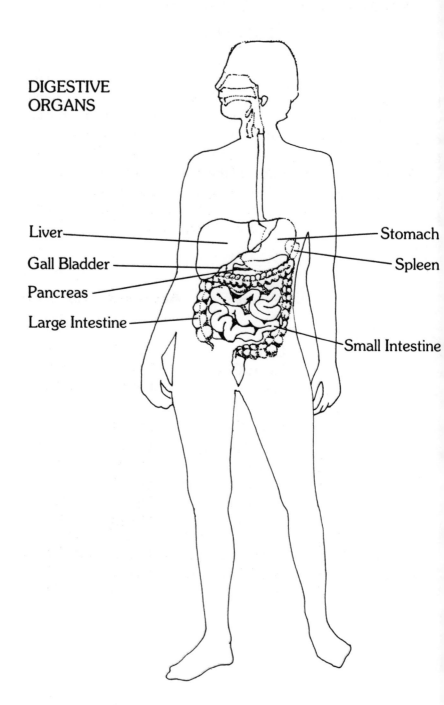

Liver

Gall Bladder

Pancreas

Large Intestine

Stomach

Spleen

Small Intestine

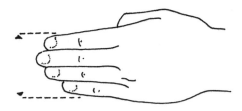

Touch Diagnosis

Shiatsu has a unique aspect of acting as both treatment and diagnostic tool. Pain and tenderness of a point or an area tells us that imbalance exists in that location. That hand, arm or leg which is painful to the touch can also inform of internal problems that already trouble you or have the potential to create trouble in the future. For example, soreness on the inside ankle of women refers to menstrual trouble. Treating this area helps to relieve period cramps and pain.

The purpose of shiatsu is to create balance and to make people whole, for that reason we are not concerned with minute detail or individual acupoints. However, certain acupoints have been used traditionally with very good results, and you may find their names and functions interesting. To a large degree our common sense and intuition would give us this information if we continued to develop our own techniques long enough.

Point locations are derived by measurements based on body ratios. The most commonly used measurement is the "body inch", which is the distance of the width of the thumb at its widest point. The four fingers together are considered three "body inches."

KEY:

Lung	=	LU		Heart	=	HT
Large Intestine	=	LI		Small Intestine	=	SI
Stomach	=	ST		Urinary Bladder	=	UB
Spleen	=	SP		Kidney	=	KD

English		Acupoint Number	Chinese
Hundred Meetings		1. GV 20	Baihui
Sun		2. extra	Taiyang
Seal Hall		3. extra	Yintang
Welcome Fragrance		4. LI 20	Yingxiang
Shielding Wind		5. TH 17	Yifeng
Wind Pond		6. GB 20	Fengchi

Heart Governer	=	HG		Conception Vessel	=	CV
Triple Heater	=	TH		Governing Vessel	=	GV
Gall Bladder	=	GB				
Liver	=	LV				

Diagnosis	Locations
atigue, weakness, spiritual point-universal energy enters the body here. Hemorroids.	Midpoint of the line connect ing the two tops of the ears.
fatigue, eye problems, headaches	In the depression in the temple.
fatigue, eye problems, headaches, regulates neural energy	Midway between the two eyebrows.
sinus, allergies, stuffy nose. Contracts mucus membranes and opens up sinus passages.	Outer border of the nose.
ear, hearing, face pain.	Back of the ear-lobe, in a depression.
colds headache, dizziness, stiff neck	In the depressions, off the mid-line of the neck, below the skull.

English	Acupoint Number	Chinese
Shoulder Well	7. GB 21	Jianjing
Crooked Pool	8. LI 11	Quchi
Arm's Three Miles	9. LI 10	Shousanli
Adjoining Valleys	10. LI 4	Hegu
Exhaustion's Palace	11. HG 8	Laogong
Yin Tomb Spring	12. SP 9	Yinlingqu
Yang Tomb Spring	13. GB 34	Yanglingq

Diagnosis	Locations
stiff neck, shoulder pain	Midway between the shoulder bone and the large vertebrae of the spine at C7.
throat, eye, tooth pain, fever	With the arm bent, midline in the crease.
face and arm problems, tones up body	Two "inches" below LI 11.
colds, headache, general body pain, whole body strengthener, with constipation the left hand point will be much tighter then the right, refers to descending colon.	At the highest point of the muscle when the thumb and the index finger are brought close together.
hand and heart pain, mental problems, painful when you are run down	In the middle of the palm between the middle and ring fingers.
menstrual and bladder problems	In the depression on the lower border just below the knee on the inside of the leg.
digestive and liver trouble	In the depression on the outside of the leg just below the knee.

English		Acupoint Number	Chinese
Leg Three Miles		14. ST 36	Zusanli
Three Yin Junction		15. SP 6	Sanyinjiao
Grandpa's Grandson		16. SP 4	Gongsun
Great Pouring		17. LV 3	Taichong
Kunlun Mountains		18. UB 60	Kunlun
Great Creek		19. KD 3	Taixi
Gushing Spring		20. KD 1	Yongquan

Diagnosis	Locations
digestion and general body tonic	Three "inches" below the indentations of the knee on the outside.
digestion, menstrual trouble, relaxes uterine muscles	Three "inches" above the tip of the inside ankle bone.
stomachache, menstruation, ankle pain, if blue blood vessels show, the pancreas is not working well, generally from too much sugar.	In a depression on the inside of the foot near the arch.
dizziness, liver trouble, insomnia	Between the first and second toe, two "inches" above the web.
headache, stiff neck, kidney/bladder trouble	On the outside of the ankle near the bone.
menses, kidney/bladder problems	On the inside of the ankle near the bone.
hypertension, stones, kidney weakness	On the sole of the foot in the depression between the second and third toes.

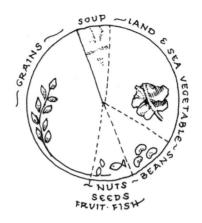

Diet and Your Health

Macrobiotics is a unique blend of Eastern and Western influences. It is a way of life according to the largest possible view. Macrobiotic principles offer a unifying way to look at nature, a way to see the universe as a whole. The practice of macrobiotics is the understanding and practical application of this natural order to our lifestyle. This includes our daily eating as well as our outlook on life.

Macrobiotic dietary principles take into account differing needs according to climate, geography, age, sex and level of activity. Our native intuition should guide us in our food choices. The practice of macrobiotics helps to develop intuition.

The dietarty link between physical, emotional and behavioral illness is becoming clear. After much investigation the National Academy of Science stated that sixty percent of all illness is diet related. It is therefore preventable. They recommend changes in our current eating patterns with a reduction of fats, sugars, refined foods and salt; with an increase in whole foods, such as fruits, vegetables and grains.

A similar connection was made over two thousand five hundred years ago. This was stated in ancient Chinese medical textbooks. It is expressed clearly in the Five Transformations chart. Various foods have specific effects on internal organs. The simplest response to the question, "What should I eat?", is 'follow traditional eating patterns. Eat whole food in its growing season."

Food can be divided into two basic divisions. Emphasize the beneficial foods and minimize as much as possible the harmful list. Your physical strength and attitude come from food. The quality of your shiatsu technique reflects your condition. Eat well and guide others toward a happier physical and emotional life.

HARMFUL FOODS

1. **Beef and other red meats.**
   High fat content, high cholesterol, excessive protein (uric acid toxemia and gout), artificial growth hormones, antibiotics. Linked to heart and vessel diseases.

2. **Poultry.**
   Same as beef and red meats, however less amounts of fat and cholesterol.

3. **Dairy products - cheese, milk, yogurt, ice cream, cottage cheese, kefir, butter and cream.**
   High fat content, excessive protein, appropriate food for nursing calves, lactose difficult for humans to digest, linked to iron deficiency anemia, fatigue syndromes and allergies.

4. **Sugar, honey, artificial sweeteners and soda pop.**
   Linked to dental caries, high blood pressure, ulcers, pancreas inability to stabilize blood sugar levels, depression, confusion, irritability, expands and weakens organs and blood vessels.

5. **Artificial and refined foods.**
   As unnatural food sources the body is unable to process properly.

BENEFICIAL FOODS

1. **Whole Cereal Grains and their products.**
   Whole wheat, brown rice, millet, corn, buckwheat, rye, barley, oats.

2. **Beans and Peas.**
   Garbanzo, lentils, aduki, black, navy, pinto, etc.

3. **Root Vegetables.**
   Carrots, onions, turnips parsnips, burdock etc.

   Ground Vegetables.
   Pumpkin, squashes, broccoli, cauliflower, etc.

   Green Leafy Vegetables.
   Kale, cabbage, watercress, mustard, etc.

4. **Seaweeds.**
   Hiziki, arame, kombu, wakame, dulse, nori, sea palm, etc.

5. **Fermented Foods.**
   Miso, soy sauce, pickles, sauerkraut, etc.

6. **Fish.**

7. **Seeds, nuts and fruits.**

About the Author

Patrick McCarty has studied Natural Health techniques for 20 years and has counseled in Macrobiotic Shiatsu since 1977. He received training in Oriental Medicine at the Shanghai College of Traditional Chinese Medicine. He is a certified shiatsu instructor and practitioner recognized by the American Oriental Bodywork Therapy Association (AOBTA). Patrick co-authored two books with Shizuko Yamamoto, *The Shiatsu Handbook* and *Whole Health Shiatsu*. He co-directs the East-West Center for Macrobiotics, a natural health education center in northern California. He is co-founder and editor of the International Macrobiotic Shiatsu Society's newsletter "Healthways." He and his wife, Meredith McCarty, travel extensively to give workshops in alternative health and to sponsor learning vacations.

SHELBYVILLE-SHELBY COUNTY
PUBLIC LIBRARY

Index

Massage, basis of, 2
Meat, health and, 53
Meridians. *See* Channels.
Movement, health and, 13

Physical activity, health and, 13

Seal Hall, 46
Sex, 14
Shiatsu
   acupoints and, 3, 4–10, 43
   back, 27–30
   back side, 20–23
   Back-shu
   breathing and, 13
   diagnosing with, 45
   disease prevention and, 3
   elements of, 19
   face down, 24–26
   foot and leg, 36–39
   front side, 30–32
   hand and arm, 33–36
   head and face, 39–42
   meaning of, 2
Shielding Wind, 46

Shoulder Well, 48
Sleep, effects on mood, 14
Small intestine, energy channels for, 6
Spleen, energy channels for, 4
Stomach, energy channels for, 5
Sun, 46
Sweeteners, health and, 53

Three Yin Junction, 50
Triple heater, energy channels for, 8

Urinary Bladder, energy channels for, 7

Welcome Fragrance, 46
Wind Pond, 46

Yamamoto, Shizuko, 1
Yang, forces of, 3, 11–12
Yang Tomb Spring, 48
Yin, forces of, 3, 11–12
Yin Tomb Spring, 48